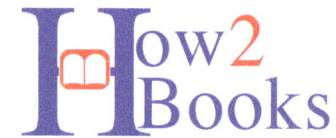

www.how2books.com.au

Your Shopping Handbook

DEVILS IN FOOD Additives

Your Shopping Handbook

Christine Thompson-Wells

Disclaimer

This is not a medical book and should not be used as such. The contents have been developed through observational theory and research (observational psychology).

The diagrams are for information and to enhance the meaning of the written text.

Statements, information and ideas within this book are for education purposes only. The text presented allows the reader to draw their own conclusions on the content offered.

Always consult with your doctor for possible illness or underlying illness.

Before dietary investigation, consult a dietician with an interest in food intolerance or food related diseases and disorders.

Information is drawn from scientific literature, web search and personal enquiry. While all care is taken, the information is not warranted as accurate. Additive numbers, E Numbers and ISN numbers are continually changing and being updated. At the time of writing this book, the Additive Numbers were current.

Christine Thompson-Wells and Books For Reading On Line.Com cannot be held liable for any errors or omissions.

ISBN 978-0-64-516124-3

*Respect for our food has been lost.
It's now time to have that respect back into our life force.
Respect for food is paramount for individual good health and the wellbeing for all people.
Food manufacturers have been dictating to the consumer, through bright and gimmicky advertising, to sell their products through visual appeal that does not always represent the quality and goodness of the product portrayed on its packaging image.
It's now time for honesty of the product and ingredients in the food we eat.*

How to work with this handbook:

Traffic light signals indicate the additives health benefit, the health caution or the health poison or toxin.

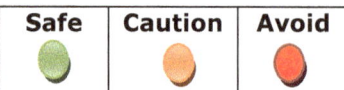

Devils: Colours (100 range)

Additive Number	Additive traffic light	Additive name	Description
100	🟢 🟠	Curcumin or turmeric	Originally a member of the ginger family. Can be artificially and synthetically produced. Very high doses of synthetic additive can cause nausea and migraines.
101	🟢 🟠	Riboflavin(i) (ii) (iii)	Riboflavin (i) is a synthetic. Can be genetically modified.
102	🔴	Tartrazine	A food colour derived from coal tar. Is used in breakfast cereals, butter, margarine and other food. Contributes to learning and behavioural

103		Alkanet or Alkannin	problems. Not allowed in some parts of the Western world. In sensitive asthmatics it may increase a reaction and hyperactivity in some children.
104		Quinoline yellow	Is an artificial coal tar dye used in the production of some food. Found in ices and ice cream and other food.
110		Sunset yellow FCF	Is a synthetic colour used in cereals, drinks, sweets and confectionary, commercially baked bakery products, and other food. May cause hyperactivity, and kidney tumours.
120		Cochineal or carmines or carmic acid	Extracted from crushed carcasses of the female Dactylopius coccus scale insect. Used in commercially baked breads and bakery products. Causes allergies, reactions for asthmatics

122	●	**Azorubine or carmoisine, C114720**	Synthetic food dye derivative of coal tar. Used in confectionary, jelly crystals and marzipan. Carcinogen, mutagen, skin rashes, hyperactivity.
123	●	**Amaranth**	Synthetic dye derived from coal tar. Found in ice cream, jams and other food. May cause birth defects. Hyperactivity. Linked to cancer.
124	●	**Ponceau 4R**	Synthetic food colour. Used in dessert toppings, colour salami, fruit pie fillings, cake mixes and other food. Causes behavioural problems, hyperactivity, learning difficulties. Linked to cancer.
127	●	**Erythrosine**	Cherry-pink/red synthetic coal tar dye. Found cocktail glacé tinned cherries, canned fruit and other food. May produce hyperactivity in children.

129		Allura red AC	Used in many sweets, confectionery, drinks, condiments and other food. Reaction by asthmatics. Linked to cancer.
132		Indigotine	Synthetic coal tar dye. Mixture of indoxyl of sodium phenylglycinate and caustic soda. Used in ice cream, sweets, and other food. Causes blood pressure. Breathing problems.
133		Brilliant blue FCF	Aluminium solution or ammonium salts. Is an artificial food colouring. Used in ice blocks, candy floss. Suspect carcinogen and Hyperactivity.
140		Chlorophyll	May be extracted by the use of dangerous solvents.
141		Chlorophyll-copper complexs (i) (ii)	High in salicylates and amines, May be extracted with dangerous solvents.

142	🔴	**Green S**	Green synthetic coal tar dye found in gravy and gravy granules, ice cream and other foods. Contributes to anger and sleeping difficulties.
143	🔴	**Fast green FCF**	An organic salt which is poorly absorbed by the intestines. Found in bakery products and other food. Allergic reactions.
150a	🔴	**Caramel I**	Produced from sugar and glucose May be made from genetically modified starches by the use of caustic. Used in biscuits, soy sauce and other foods and cola. Linked to birth defects and some neurological disorders.
150b	🔴	**Caramel II Sulfite caramel**	Made from sucrose in the presence of ammonia, ammonium sulphate, sulphur dioxide or sodium hydroxide. Used in tea, snacks and other foods. Causes hyperactivity, gastrointestinal conditions and poor health.

150c	●	Caramel III Ammonia process	Contains ammonia. Used in confectionary, gravy, BBQ sauce and other foods. May cause hyperactivity, liver problems. Linked to ADHD.
150d	●	Caramel IV Amonia sulphite process	Known as 4-Mel is a sulfite ammonia. Used in fizzy drinks, baked good, chocolate and other foods. Is linked to asthma, hyperactivity and other health problems.
151	●	Brilliant black BN or Brilliant black PN	A synthetic, black tar derivative used in brown sauces, black current cake mixes and other foods. Causes hyperactivity and linked to cancer
153	●	Carbons black or Vegetable carbon	Is black in colour and may be derived from animal or vegetable carbon. Used in health foods, liquorice, sweets. Linked to cancer.

155		**Brown HT also called chocolate brown HT, C1 52028**	Synthetic coal tar diazo dye. Used to substitute cocoa. Used in chocolate, ice cream and other foods. Causes hyperactivity and asthma sensitivity.
160a		**Carotene**	Synthetic carotene is extracted by the dangerous solvent hexane. Proven to cause birth defects.
160c		**Paprica**	Is a natural food extract that can be extracted through dangerous solvents. Linked to cancer
160d		**Lycopene**	Natural Lycopene has been proven to be a powerful anti-cancer agent. If possible, check for extraction methods.
160e		**Betta-apo-8'-Carotenal (30)**	If extracted with hexane may cause severe sickness. Used in cheeses and other food.
160f		**Betta-apo-8' Carotenoic acid, methyl or ethyl ester (30)**	May be a synthetic colour extracted from beta-carotene with dangerous solvents, including hexane. Linked to endocrine disturbance.

161a	🟡 🔴	Flavoxanthin	May cause headaches. On alert in the US and the European Union.

161b	🟡 🔴	Lutein	Found in green leaves and egg yolks. May be extracted through the use of dangerous chemicals.

161c	🟡	Kryptoxanthin or Cryptoxanthin	Is extracted from flower petals and bovine serum. On alert in the US and European Union.

161d	🟡	Rubixanthin	Extracted from rose hips. Can be extracted with dangerous hexane

161e	🟡 🔴	Violoxanthin	Derived from a number of different plants including pansies. Check for method of extraction.

161f	🟡	Rhodoxanthin	Found in small quantities in a variety of plants and some bird feathers. On alert in the US and the European Union.

162		Beet red	Used in meat burgers, ice cream, jellies and other foods. Linked to tumours, cancer, blood disorders.
163		Anthocyanins or grape skin or blackcurrent extract	Derived from plants and flowers. Used in soups, confectionary and other foods. Safe if extracted without hexane.
164		Saffron or Crocetin or crocin, also known as gardenia yellow	Can be mixed with synthetic or artificial colour. Can cause hypersensitive reactions.
170		Calcium carbonate also calcium carbonate (i) and (ii)	Used in toothpaste, white paint and cleaning powders. Used in bread, cakes and other foods. Contributes to confused behaviour and other health problems.
171		Titanium dioxide	Used in vitamin supplements, biscuits and other food. Linked to cell death, cancer and other health conditions.

172	○ ○	Iron oxide also Iron oxide (i) (ii) (iii)	Used to colour capsules and health food vitamins also used herbal supplements. Also used in cake mixes and other food. May lead to kidney stones and other health concerns.
173	○	Aluminium	There's no dietary requirement for this additive to be put into and food or drink product. Used in chocolate and other foods. Is linked to Parkinson's disease and other health problems.
174	○	Silver	Is used as a colouring food agent in chocolate and food decoration. May cause lung and kidney damage.
175	○	Gold	Gold has no dietary requirements within the human body. Used in cake decoration. Severe allergic reactions.

180	●	Lithol rupine BK	Derived from coal tar and petroleum. Used in cheese rind. Can cause hyperactivity in children.
181	● ●	Tannic acid Tannins	Can be natural or synthetic. Used in tea and coffee. Can cause liver damage and other health problems.

Devils: Preservatives (200 range)

200	●	Sorbic acid	Can be natural or synthetic. Used in yogurt, soft drinks and other food. Is linked to hyperactivity and behavioural problems, liver damage and cancer.
201	●	Sodium sorbate	Synthetic preservative used in yogurt, cheeses and other food. Asthmatics avoid, causes liver damage and other health problems.
202	●	Potassium sorbate	A synthetic additive used in concentrated fruit juices, jams and other foods. Can cause liver damage and stomach discomfort.

203	🔴	Calcium sorbate	Chemical preservative used in fruit juice, margarine and other foods. Causes skin irritation and allergic reactions.
210	🔴	Benzoic acid	A resin used in margarine, fruit juices and other food. Can cause hyperactivity, neurological disorders and other health problems.
211	🔴	Sodium benzoate	A chemical synthetic used to disguise poor taste. Used in fruit juices, meat products and other food. Linked to ADHD, cancer and other health problems.
212	🔴	Potassium benzoate	A synthetic preservative used in cheesecake mix, soft drinks and other foods. Can contribute to behavioural problems, depression and health problems.

213	●	Calcium benzoate	A food additive commonly used in fruit juice, bread making and other foods. Asthmatics avoid. Can contribute to neurological disorders and health problems.
216	● ●	Sodium propyl p-hydroxyben-zoate	A synthetic powder used in fruit sauces, fruit desserts and other foods. Can cause problems for asthmatics.
218	●	Methylpara-ben or methyl-p-hydroxyben-zoate	Used as a preservative in baked goods. Added to milk and other foods. Causes anger, hormone disruption and other health concerns.
220	●	Sulphur dioxide	A preservative obtained from coal tar. Used in beer, juices, potato products and other foods and drink. Can cause facial swelling and other health concerns.

221	●	Sodium sulphite, sulfite	Is a sulphite additive used in fruit drinks, sausages and other foods. Can cause intestinal disorders, behavioural problems.
222	●	Sodium hydrogen bisulphite, bisulfite	A synthetic preservative used in corn syrup, milk, custards and other foods. Can contribute to genetic damage, swelling of the brain and other health concerns.
223	●	Sodium metabisul-phate	A bleaching agent and preservative used in cracker biscuits, tomato juice and other foods. Can cause respiratory reactions, behavioural problems and other health concerns.
224	●	Potassium metabisul-phite	Used as a bleaching agent in dried fruits, chips or crisps and in other foods. Can cause behavioural problems, seizures and other health problems.

225		Potassium sulphite (also called potash of sulphur) (SOP)	Is used as a bleaching agent in sugar production. Can cause behavioural problems and ADHD.
234		Nisin	An additive used to extend shelf life in meat, cheeses and other foods. Asthmatics should avoid. May cause other health problems.
235		Natamycin	Used as a food preservative. Can cause vomiting, anorexia and related health conditions.
242		Dimethyl dicarbonate DMDC	A dangerous toxin found in children's juices and drinks. Can cause breathing problems if inhaled.
243		Ethyl lauroyl arginate	Concentrated forms can be dangerous. Used in fruit drinks and meat products. Can cause breathing difficulties and other health issues.

249	●	**Potassium nitrite**	A common preservative used worldwide. Used to colour meat and fish. Can contribute to behavioural problems, cancer and other health problems.
250	●	**Sodium nitrite**	A dangerous chemical used in ham, bacon and other foods. Contributes to stomach cancer, Parkinson's disease and other health conditions.
251	●	**Sodium nitrate Chile saltpetre**	A mineral used in curing meat. Can contributes to asthma, learning difficulties, cancer and other health problems.
252	●	**Potassium nitrate**	An additive that may be derived from waste vegetable matter. Used in frankfurters, cheeses and other foods. Can contribute to asthma, dizziness and other health conditions.

Code			Name	Description
260	🟠	🔴	**Acetic acid glacial**	A synthetic additive. Is used as a flavour enhancer in pickles, chutneys and other foods. Can cause asthma and allergic reactions.
261	🟠	🔴	**Potassium acetate or potassium diacetate (i) (ii)**	A food acid regulator. Used in pickles and vinegar. Will aggravate food intolerances.
262	🟠	🔴	**Sodium acetate Sodium diacetate (i) (ii)**	Food acidity regulator used in snack foods, potato chips and other foods. Can contribute to intestinal upset and severe reactions.
263	🟠	🔴	**Calcium acetate**	Made from wood alcohol. Used as a regulator in cake mixes, thickening agents. Can cause nausea, vomiting and other health concerns.
270	🟠	🔴	**Lactic acid**	Is used in fermented milk, infant milk, cheeses and other food products. Not suitable for babies.

280	●	Propionic acid	Can be commercially made from carbon monoxide. Used in some breads and dough products. Linked to cancer.
281	●	Sodium propionate	A synthetic preservative. Used in processed cheese, bread and other food products. Can cause shortness in breath. May be linked to cancer.
282	●	Calcium propionate	Is a dangerous synthetic preservative. Used in breads and biscuits manufacture. Linked to ADHD. Severe allergic reactions.
283	●	Potassium propionate	Is a dangerous synthetic preservative. Used in pastries, biscuits and other food products. Can cause gastro intestinal upset and other health problems.

290		Carbon dioxide	An acidity regulator. Use in fizzy and soft drinks. Is linked to impaired fertility and other health concerns.
296		Malic acid	In commercial food production is used as a synthetic acidity regulator. Used in jams and drinks. Can contribute to upset stomach and other health conditions.
297		Fumaric acid	Used as an acidity regulator. A raising agent in bread and cakes. Can cause adverse allergy reactions.

Devils: Antioxidants (300 range)

300		Ascorbic acid Vitamin C	Can be synthetically made from genetically modified crops. Added to breakfast cereals, tinned baby food. Can cause vomiting, diarrhoea and other health concerns.

301	red	Sodium ascorbate	Is synthetic used as an antioxidant in breads and cooked food, Can cause swelling of the tongue and face.
302	green, orange	Calcium ascorbate	Is used as an antioxidant and preservative. Used in bouillons and other food products.
303	orange, red	Potassium ascorbate	Used in dairy-based drinks, processed cheese and other foods. Can lead to mood swings and other health concerns.
304	green	Ascorbyl palmitate	Combined with palmitate and ascorbic acid.
307	orange	α-Tocopherol or vitamin E	A synthetic vitamin E. Used in margarine and some other oils. On alert in the United States, European Union, New Zealand and Australia
307b	orange	Tocopherols concentrate, mixed	Synthetic vitamin E. On alert in the United States.

308		α-Tocopherol - synthetic	As 307, 307b

309		γ-Tocopherol-synthetic	As 307b and 308

310		Propyl gallate	Is a synthesised additive. Used in margarine. Can cause allergic reactions, is linked to cancer.

311		Octyl gallate	Derived from nut galls. Used in dairy and other foods. Can cause hyperactivity and insomnia.

315		Erythorbic acid	A synthetic antioxidant. Used in dairy-based drinks and cheeses.

316		Sodium erythorbate	A synthetic antioxidant used in meat and poultry. Side effects: headaches, body flushes.

319		tert-Butylhydro-quinone (TBHQ)	A dangerous additive derived from petroleum. Used in oils and margarines. Severe allergic reactions.

320	🔴	Butylated hydroxyanisole (BHA)	Derived from petroleum. Used in soft drinks, biscuits and other foods. Can cause hyperactivity. Linked to liver damage. Banned in some countries.
321	🔴	Butylated hydroxyto-luene	Is a petroleum derivative and synthetic antioxidant. Used in biscuits, cakes and other foods. Causes hyperactivity, learning difficulties and other health conditions.
322	🟢 🟠	Lecithin also lecithin (i) (ii)	Is commercially synthesised. Methods of extraction should be considered. Used in margarine, ice cream and other food products.

Devils: More food acids (300 range)

325	🟠 🔴	Sodium lactate (food acid)	Used as an acidity regulator. Used in cakes, cheeses and other foods. May cause chest pain, wheezing and other health conditions.

326	● ●	Potassium lactate	May be genetically modified from pork. Used in cheeses, ice cream and other foods. Not recommended for children.
327	●	Calcium lactate	Acidity regulator extracted from milk. Used in condensed milk. May give adverse reactions to babies.
328	● ●	Ammonium lactate	Acidity regulator used in sweets, cakes and other foods. Not safe for babies.
329	● ●	Magnesium lactate DL	Acidity regulator used in flour treatment. May cause stomach bloating. Not recommended for babies.
330	●	Citric acid	Acidity regulator. In commercial production contains PFGA 620. Used in jams, sweets and other foods. Can cause eating disorders and other health conditions.

331	🔴	Sodium dihydrogen citrate (ii) Disodium monohydrogen citrate (iii) Trisodium citrate	Synthesized additive used in marmalades, ice cream and other foods. May cause intestinal upset and other health conditions
332	🟡 🔴	Potassium citrate and Potassium dihydrogen citrate (i) Tripotassium citrate (ii)	Synthetic acidity regulator used in soft drinks. On alert in the United States.
333	🟡 🔴	Calcium citrate Monsodium citrate (i) Dicalcium citrate (ii) Tricalcium citrate (iii)	Synthesized acidity regulator. Used in ice cream, jams and other foods. May contribute to arthritic symptoms and/or liver problems.
334	🟡 🔴	Tartaric acid	Synthesized additive used in dried egg whites, bakery products and other food. Can cause allergic reactions and intestinal problems.

335		Sodium tartrate (i) Monsodium tartrate (ii) Disodium tartrate	Commercially synthesized used in baking powder, margarine and other foods. Can contribute to stomach cramps, kidney conditions and other health issues.
336		Potassium tartrates or Potassium acid tartrates (i) Monopotassium tartrate (ii) Dipotassium tartrate	Used as an acidity regulator in lollies, jams and other foods. Can interfere with blood pressure and aggravate intestinal function.
337		Sodium potassium tartrates	Is a mineral salt found in most commercially produced foods. Used in cola drinks, cheese and other foods.
338		Phosphoric acid	Derived from phosphate ore, used as an acidity regulator. Used in cola, processed meats and other foods. Can lead to digestive disorders, osteoporosis and other health condtions.

25

Devils: Mineral salts (300 range)

339	●	Sodium phosphates (i) Sodium dihydrogen phosphate (ii) Disodium hydrogen phosphate (iii) Trisodium phosphate	Produced from animal bone or mined. Used as an anti-caking agent in baked goods, cola drinks and other food. Linked to kidney disease and other health conditions.
340	●	Potassium phosphate, dibasic (i) Potassium dihydrogen phosphate (ii) Dipotassium hydrogen phosphate (iii) Tripotassium phosphate	Produced from animal bones or mined. Used as an antioxidant in drinking chocolate, milk and other foods. Linked to kidney stones, heart arrhythmia and other health conditions.
341	● ●	Calcium phosphate (i) Calcium dihydrogen phosphate (ii) Calcium hydrogen phosphate (iii) Tricalcium phosphate	Used as an anti-caking agent in bread, breakfast cereals and other foods. Linked to digestive disorders and tissue damage.

342	●	**Ammonium phosphates (i) Ammonium dihydrogen phosphate (ii) Diammonium hydrogen phosphate**	In commercial production, ammonium is used to dissolve the rock. Is used in flour and the purification of sugar.
343	●	**Magnesium phosphate (i) Magnesium dihydrogen phosphate (ii) Magnesium hydrogen phosphate (iii) Trimagnesium phosphate**	Used as an anti-caking agent. Derived from animal bones or mined. Used in commercially baked products, food supplements and other foods.
349	●	**Ammonium malate**	Is an ammonium salt used in soft drinks, confectionary and other foods. On alert in the United States and the European Union.

350		Sodium hydrogen malate (i) Sodium hydrogen DL – malate (ii) Sodium DL malate	Used as a low salt substitute. Used in fruit drinks, dairy blends. Possibly harmful for the human system and brain. On alert in the United States, European Union, New Zealand and Australia.
351		Potassium malates (i) Potassium hydrogen malate (ii) Potassium malate	In commercial production is a synthesized additive. Used in fruit drinks, jams and other foods. On alert in the United States, European Union, New Zealand and Australia.
352		Calcium malate (i) Calcium hydrogen malate (ii) Calcium malate, D, L-	Used as a thickener in ice cream, fried products and other foods. Not allowed in foods for infants. On alert in the United States.
353		Metatartaric acid	Not allowed in infants or young children's food.

354		Calcium tartrate	Is used as a food modifying agent. Used in infant rusks. Not recommended for infants. May cause gastro-enteritis in adults.
355		Adipic acid	Synthetic additive derived from petroleum and hexane. Used as a food flavouring in fruit juices, ice blocks and other foods. Causes nausea, delayed growth and other health problems.
357		Potassium adipate	In commercial food production, is extracted using petroleum and hexane. Used as a gelling agent in fruit juices, jams and other foods. Can lead to tissue damage and heart arrhythmia.
359		Ammonium adipates	Is ammonium salt used in fermented milks, cheese and in other foods. On alert in the United States and the European Union.

363	●	Succinic acid	Used as a growth inhibitor in breads, contributes to allergies and other health conditions. Banned in many countries.
365	● ●	Sodium fumarate	Used as a food acid regulator in bakery products, egg whites and other food. Can cause kidney damage and other health conditions. On alert in the United States and the European Union.
366	● ●	Potasium fumerate	Regulates acidity in jams and preserves. More research into this product is required.
367	● ●	Calcium fumerate	Used as a food additive in commercial products. Added to dietary supplements. Not permitted in the European Union.
368	● ●	Ammonium fumerate	Food regulator used in tortillas and other food products. On alert in the United States. Not permitted in the European Union.

380	●	Tri-ammonium citrate	In commercial production is a synthesized food regulator. Used in dietary supplements, chocolate and other foods. Linked to nerve cell destruction and other health conditions.
381	●	Ferric ammonium citrate	Is a synthetic caking agent regulator. Used in breakfast cereals and other foods. On alert in the European Union.
385	●	Calcium disodium ethylene-diaminete-traacetate or calcium disodium EDTA	Is a synthetic food antioxidant used in soft drinks, mayonnaise and other foods. Can contribute to muscle cramps, cancer and other health conditions.

Devils: Vegetable gums, thickeners, stabilisers, emulsifiers and glazing agents (400 range)

400	🟡 🔴	**Alginic acid**	A natural product from brown seaweed. Used as a thickening agent in ice cream, cheeses and other food products. Linked to severe allergic reactions and neurological disorders.
401	🟡 🔴	**Sodium alginate**	In commercial food production is used as a bulking agent in dairy products, processed meats and other foods. May be linked to birth defects and severe allergic reaction.
402	🟡 🔴	**Potassium alginate**	In commercial food manufacture is used as bulking agent. Used in thickened cream, custards and other foods. May be linked to birth defects, neurological disorders and other health conditions.

403	●●	Ammonium alginate	Is used as a bulking agent in custard mixes, jams and other foods. May cause allergic reaction. Can affect the gastrointestinal tract.
404	●●	Calcium alginate	An emulsifier derived from seaweed. Used in custard powders, ice cream and other foods. May be linked to severe allergic reactions and other health problems.
405	●	Propylene glycol alginate	Extracted from brown seaweed by petroleum extraction. Used in marmalade, ice cream and other foods. May cause neurological disorders. Banned in France.
406	●●	Agar or agar agar	Derived from seaweed. Used in meringues, yogurt and other foods. Causes flatulence and linked to cancer.

Number	Color	Name	Description
407	🔴	Carrageenan	Fibre extracted from seaweed and used as a thickener in soy milk, sauces and other food. Is linked to gastrointestinal malignancy and other bowel disorder.
409	🟢 🟠	Arabinoga-lactan or larch gum	Is extracted from larch wood. Used in bakery products, chocolate and other foods. On alert in the European Union.
410	🟠	Locust bean gum or carob bean gum	A vegetable extract from seaweed. Used in sweets, soft drinks and other foods. Can cause allergic reactions.
412	🔴	Guar gum	A food thickener and stabiliser. Used in dairy products, cheeses and other foods. Linked to intestinal disorders and cancer.
413	🔴	Tragacanth gum	Is used as an food emulsifier and stabiliser. Used in cottage cheese, ice cream and other foods. Linked to liver damage, asthma and other health conditions.

414	🟡 🔴	**Gum Arabic or Acacia gum**	Is a thickening agent used in the manufacture of marshmallows, soft drinks and other foods. Linked to severe asthma attacks, cancer and other health conditions.
415	🟡	**Xanthan Gum**	A common additive used as an emulsifies. Can be genetically modified. Used in baked goods, dairy and other foods. May contribute to stomach bloating, cramps and other discomforts.
416	🟡 🔴	**Karaya gum**	A processed vegetable gum. Used in potato and cereal-based snacks, bakery products and other foods. Is an allergen and can cause other health problems.
417	🟡 🔴	**Tara gum**	Is used as a thickener in jellies, yogurt and other foods. Can contribute to shortness of breath, tightness in the chest and other health conditions.

418	⬤⬤	Gellan gum	Is used as a gelling agent in ice cream, soy milk and other foods. Can cause abdominal bloating and excessive gas. On alert in the United States.

Devils: Humectants also used as sweeteners (400 range)

420	⬤⬤	Sorbitol or sorbitol syrup and Sorbitol (i) and(ii)	An artificial sweetener used as a bulking agent in biscuits, ice cream and other foods. Can cause gastric disturbance, kidney stones and other health conditions.
421	⬤	Mannitol	Produced commercially through hydrogenation of invert sugar. Used in baked goods, confectionary and other foods. Severe allergic reactions, kidney damage and other health problems.
422	⬤⬤	Glycerine or glycerol	A synthetic sweetener. Used in baked goods, and other foods. Can cause endocrine disruption, kidney disorders and other health conditions

Devils: Emulsifiers (400 range)

431	🔴	Polyoxy-ethylene (40) stearate	Synthetic compound and emulsifier from petroleum. Used in bread and puddings. Linked to liver damage, urinary tract problems and other health conditions.
433	🔴	Polysorbate 80 or Polyoxy-ethylene (20) sorbitan monooleate or PEG 80	A synthetic additive used in artificial flavourings. Used in cupcake, cake mixes and other foods. Can irritate respiratory tract. Linked to kidney disorders.
435	🔴	Polysorbate 60 or Polyoxy-ethylene (20) Sorbitan monostearate or Peg 60	A synthetic flavouring additive used in commercially made dough and dough products. Can cause kidney and liver damage.
436	🔴	Polysorbate 65 or Polyoxy-ethylene (20) sorbitan tristearate	A synthetic of a petrol derivative. Used in long-life milk, cake fillings and in other foods. Linked to cancer, kidney damage and other health concerns.

440	🟠🟠	Pectin	A synthetic dangerous commercial product. Used as a gelling agent in confectionary, milk and other products. Can cause intestinal problems and flatulence.
442	🟠	Ammonium salts of phosphatidic acid Soy lecithin	Synthetic can be a derivative of ammonia fatty acids. Used in chocolate, cakes and other foods. Can affect blood pressure, add to weight gain.
444	🟠	Sucrose acetate isobutyrate	A synthetic of cane sugar. Used in ice creams, cheeses and other foods. May cause respiratory and digestive problems.
445	🟠	Glycerol esters of rosin Glycerol esters of gum rosin (i) Glycerol esters of tall oil rosin (ii) Glycerol esters of wood rosins (iii)	Extracted from the solvent methanol. Used in pasteurised products including cheese, ice cream and other foods. Can cause mental confusion; can increase liver size and other health problems.

Devils: More mineral salts (400 range)

450		Diphosphates (i) Disodium diphosphate (ii) Trisodium diphosphate (iii) Tetrasodium diphosphate (iv) Dipotassium diphosphate (v) Tetrapotassium diphosphate (vi) Dicalcium diphosphate (vii) Calcium dihydrogen diphosphate (viii) Dimagnesium diphosphate (ix) Magnesium dihydrogen diphosphate	A synthetic from carbonates. Used in some bread and baked goods. Linked to kidney damage and disease and other health conditions.

451		Potassium triphosphates	Salts of animal bones or mined. Used in ham and cured meats. Can increase blood pressure, muscle spasm and other health concerns.

452	●	Potassium polymetaphos-phate (i) Sodium phosphate (ii) Potassium phosphate (iii) Sodium calcium phosphate (iv) Calcium phosphate (v) Ammonium phosphate (vi) Sodium potassium tripolypho-sphate	Is a gluten-free additive. Used as a food and drink stabiliser in canned meats, some dairy produce and other foods. Is linked to kidney damage, intestinal disorders and other health conditions.

Devils: Thickeners (400 range)

460	● ●	Cellulose microcrystal-line and cellulose powdered	Refined from wood pulp and genetically modified cotton stems. Used as an anti-caking agent in fermented milk, margarine and other foods.

461	●	Methyl cellulose	A synthetic from wood and cotton products. Is chemically modified. Used in ice cream, yoghurts and other food products. Can cause intestinal disorders, is linked to cancer.

463	🔴	Hydroxy-propyl cellulose	A synthetic additive manufactured from wood and a petroleum by-product. Is used as a thickening agent in cereals, dairy products and other foods. Can cause intestinal problems. Is linked to cancer.
464	🔴	Hydroxy-propyl methyl cellulose	A plastic and petroleum-based product. Used in baby formula, milk powders and other food and drink products. Can cause endocrine disruption, digestive problems and other health problems.
465	🔴	Methyl ethyl cellulose	A by-product of petroleum used as a thickening agent in cheaper chocolate products, ice cream and other foods. Causing bowel bloating. Is linked to cancer
466	🔴	Sodium carboxy-methyl cellulose and cellulose gum (CMC)	A by-product of petroleum used in breads, bread products, low-calorie cream and other food products. Linked to cancer.

470	🟠	**Salts of fatty acids** **Salts of aluminium, ammonia, calcium, magnesium, potassium and sodium** Also known as: **(i) Salts of myristic, palmitic and stearic acids with ammonia, calcium, potassium and sodium** **(ii) Salts of oleic acid with calcium, potassium and sodium** **(iii)Magnesium stearate**	Synthetic fatty acids used as an emulsifier in sweeteners, anti-caking agent in oven-ready chips, cake mixes and other foods. Can contribute to liver disorders, disrupt the endocrine system and contribute to other health concerns.
471	🟠	**Mono and di-glycerides of fatty acids**	Synthetic fats from pork extraction used as thickening agents, in cake mixes and other food products. Can contribute to birth defects and cancer.

472a	●	Acetic and fatty acid esters of glycerol	A synthetic additive, which may be extracted using petroleum-based chemicals. Used in pastry, baked goods and other foods. Can interfere with intestinal function, mental ability and cause other health concerns.
472b	●	Lactic and fatty acid esters of glycerol	Derived from synthetic fats. May be extracted using petroleum-based chemicals. Used in dairy foods, margarine and other food products. Can interfere with intestinal functions, cause diarrhoea and other health problems.
472c	●	Citric and fatty acid esters of glycerol	Synthetic chemical which form PFGA[1] Produced using many levels of petroleum. Used in dairy foods, batters and other manufactured food. Contributes to ADHD, facial swelling and other health conditions.

[1] Processed free glutamic acid is highly refined and unbound to amino acids

472e	🔴	Diacetyltartaric and fatty acid esters of glycerol	A dangerous synthetic additive used to make crusty bread, baked goods and other foods. May contribute to birth defects and cancer.
472f	🔴	Mixed tartaric, acetic and fatty acid esters of glycerol or tartaric, acetic and fatty acid esters of glycerol (mixed)	Mainly made from synthetic fats using petroleum-based chemicals. Used in oven-ready chips, dairy foods and other manufactured foods. Can cause mental confusion, dizziness and other health concerns.
473	🔴	Sucrose esters of fatty acids	Usually manufactured in the presence of solvents. Used in bakery goods, dairy products and other foods and drink. May cause stomach pain, linked to poisoning.
475	🟡 🔴	Polyglycerol esters of fatty acids	Poorly tested additives. Used in margarine, sponge cakes and other food products. They may pose their own problems.

476	●	Poly-glycerol esters of inter-esterified ricinoleic acid (PGPR)[2]	Is a synthetic product extracted from acetone-benzene and petroleum solution. Used in cocoa butter, commercially baked products. May cause gastrointestinal irritation, vomiting and other health concerns.
477	●	Propylene glycol mono- and di-esters or Propylene glycol esters of fatty acids	A synthetic compound that may be derived from petroleum. Found in baker products, ice cream and other foods. May cause severe reactions and a reduction in the nervous system.
480	●	Dioctyl sodium sulpho-succinate	A mixture of fatty acids and petroleum. Used in syrups to make them spread evenly, soft drinks and other foods and drinks. Can cause cramps and abdominal pain.

---

[2] PGPR is an emulsifier extracted from castor or soy bean oil.

481	Sodium lactylate i) Sodium stearoyl lactylate (ii) Sodium oleyl lactylate (SSL)	Is a soda ash. Used as a stabiliser in flour, baked goods, confectionary and in other food products. Inadequate research on this additive to date.
482	Calcium lactylate (i) Calcium stearoyl lactylate (ii) Calcium oleyl lactylate	A synthetic emulsifier used in flour, dough products, cereals and other food products. May cause Irritable Bowel Syndrome (IBS), migraine and other health concerns.
491	Sorbitan monostearate	A synthetic used as an emulsifier. Used in flavoured milk, cake mixes and other food products. Linked to eczema, kidney stones and other health conditions.
492	Sorbitan tristearate (STS)	Synthetic product increasing the absorption of fat. Used in bakery goods, marmalades and other food products. Can cause intestinal problems, ill health.

Devils: Mineral salts (often used as anti-caking agents (500 range)

500		Sodium bicar-bonate, (i) Sodium carbonate (ii) Sodium hydrogen carbonate (iii) Sodium sesqui-carbonate	A synthetic raising agent used in soft drinks, battersand other foods. Large quantities cause gastric conditions and other health issues.
501		Potassium bicarbonate, Potassium carbonate	A synthetic from potassium carbonate and carbon dioxide used in cocoa, custard powders and other foods. Will irritate the lungs.
503		Ammonium carbonates (i) Ammon-ium carbonate (ii) Ammon-ium hydrogen carbonate	An acidity regulator used in bakery, confectionary and other foods. Can cause loss of calcium, nerve destruction and other health conditions.

504		Magnesium carbonate (i) Magnesium carbonate (ii) Magnesium hydroxide carbonate	An anti-caking, bleaching and modifying agent. Used as a food additive in low-sodium substitute.
507		Hydrochloric acid HCI	A corrosive compound. Used as an acidity regulator and food enhancement in gelatine, corn flour and other food products. Can cause gastric ulceration and other health conditions.
508		Potassium chloride KCL	Used as a food enrichment additive, flavouring agent in breads, and other foods. Allergic reactions, chest pains and other health problems.
509		Calcium chloride	May contain aluminium. Used as a firming agent in chocolate, breads and other foods. Can cause intestinal ulceration and other health conditions.

510	⬤ ⬤	Ammonium chloride	Used as a bulking agent in commercial food production in breads and bread mixes. Avoid if suffering with kidney or liver conditions.
511	⬤	Magnesium chloride	Commercially produced by introducing mercury to create amalgam with sodium. Used in tofu, baby formulas and other foods. Linked to endocrine disruption.
512	⬤	Stannous chloride	Is prepared from hydrochloric acid. May be used in baby and dietary formulas and in other foods. Can cause arrhythmia and affect the nervous system.
514	⬤	Sodium sulphates (i) Sodium sulfate (ii) Sodium hydrogen sulphate or Sulphate of soda	Used as an anti-caking agent in biscuits, sweets and other foods. May affect asthmatics.

515	Potass-ium sulphates SOP (i) Potass-ium sulphate (ii) Potass-ium hydrogen sulfate	Prepared from potassium chloride and sulphuric acid. Used in the biscuits, confectionary and other foods. Linked to intestinal bleeding, kidney enlargement and other health conditions
516	Calcium sulphate Also known as: Plaster of Paris, Gypsum and Drierite	Used as a firming agent in frozen desserts, flour and bakery products and other foods. Can cause intestinal blockage, constipation and other health concerns.
518	Magnesium sulphate	Prepared from magnesium salts and sulphuric acid. May be used in infant formulas, soft drinks and in other food or in medicinal products. People with kidney disorder should avoid.

519	●	Copper II (Cupric sulphate) Also known as (Blue vitriol and bluestone)	Produced industrially by treating copper with sulphuric acid oxides. Used in meat and foods to maintain colour intensity in meat, cereals and other foods. Is a neurotoxin.
520	●	Aluminium sulphate (anhydrous)	Produced from aluminium hydroxide and sulphuric acid. Added to pickles, tap water and other foods. May contribute to liver disease.
521	●	Sodium aluminium sulphate (Soda alum or sodium alum)	Is produced from sodium and aluminium sulphates. Used in cheeses, flour products and other foods. Can cause premature senility and other health conditions.
522	●	Potassium aluminium sulphate	Manufactured from potassium and aluminium sulphates. Used in breads, cakes and other foods. May be linked to Parkinson's and related diseases.

523	●	Aluminium ferric ammonium sulphate	Produced from aluminium sulphate and ammonium sulphate. Is used in baking powder and as a food colour stabiliser. Used in commercial bakeries. Linked to Alzheimer's and related diseases.
524	●	Aluminium ferric ammonium sulphate, Aluminium-ammonium	Sodium hydroxide, a highly corrosive additive. Used in tinned vegetables, sour cream and other food products. Can cause adverse reactions, shock and death.
525	●	Potassium hydroxide Potassium lye or Caustic potash	A mineral toxic, highly corrosive caustic salt. Used in cocoa, black olives and other food products. Can cause vomiting, shock and other health concerns.
526	●	Calcium hydroxide	A product of lime used as a firming and acidity regulator. Used in cocoa, jams and other foods. Can contribute to tissue damage, rupture of blood cells and other health concerns.

529		Calcium oxide (Quick lime)	A mineral salt used in many types of bread and food products. Is highly corrosive and toxic. May be safe in small quantities.
530		Magnesium oxide	Used in the food industry as an anti-caking agent. Used in canned peas, cocoa and other foods. Causes weakness and tiredness. Banned in some countries.
535		Sodium ferrocyanide Also known as (Yellow prussiate of soda)	Produced industrially from hydrogen cyanide. Used as an anti-caking agent. Harmful to the human body.
536		Potassium ferrocyanide (Yellow prussiate of potash)	A by-product of coal and gas production. Contains cyanide. Used in seasonings and spices. Reduces the transportation of oxygen to the blood.

537	●	Ferrous hexacyano-manganate	Manufactuered from mangano-cyanide. Used as an anti-caking agent and in the manufacture of liquorice. On alert in the United States.
538	●	Calcium ferrocyanide	A synthetic additive manufactured from ferrocyanide, hydrogen and calcium hydroxide. Used in seasonings and spices. May cause breathing difficulties, headaches and other health problems.
539	●	Sodium thiosulphate	Produced from liquid waste. Used to prevent browning in manufactured potato products. On alert in the European Union.
540	●	Dicalcium diphosphate or (Acid calcium phosphate)	Used as a food additive in dietary supplements, breakfast cereals and other foods. May lead to osteoporosis and other like diseases.

541	🔴	**Sodium aluminium phosphates** **(i) Sodium aluminium phosphate, acidic** **(i) Sodium aluminium phosphate, basic**	A synthetic additive produced from sodium hydroxide, aluminium and phosphoric acid. Used in baked goods, cheese and other foods. Is linked to Parkinson's and like diseases.
542	🟠 🔴	**Bone phosphate**	Produced from steaming degreased bones of pigs and cattle. Used as an anti-caking agent in dried milk for coffee machines. On alert in the United States.
551	🟢 🟠	**Silicon dioxide, amorphous (Silica)**	Derived from sand. Used as an anti-caking agent and thickener in dried milk, sausages and other foods.
552	🟢 🟠	**Calcium silicate**	Can be a synthetic. Used as an anti-caking agent. Used in dried eggs, baking powder and other food stuffs. Further research needed.

553	●	i) Magnes-ium silicate (i) Magnes-ium trisilicate (iii) talc	A synthetic additive used as an anti-caking agent. Used as a dusting powder on rice, chocolate and other foods. May be linked to cancer, kidney disease and other health conditions.
554	●	Sodium alumina-silicaate	A synthetic neurotoxin used as a food additive in the global food industry. Used as an anti-caking agent in dried milk and other foods. May cause headaches, rheumatism and other health conditions.
555	●	Potassium aluminium silicate	Partly produced from aluminium is a neurotoxic used as an anti-caking agent in dried milk, flours and other food products. May contribute to Alzheimer's and other like diseases.

556	🔴	**Calcium aluminium silicate**	Contains aluminium, a neurotoxin. Used as an anti-caking agent in milk powders, egg mixes and other foods. Causes bone loss, stomach problems and other health conditions.
558	🟢 🟠	**Bentonite**	A natural clay which can be ingested. Used as an anti-caking agent. In some instances used in the food industry in cereals.
559	🔴	**Aluminium silicate (Kaolin)**	Manufactured from aluminium oxide. Used as an anti-caking agent in dried milk for coffee machines. Is linked to kidney and bowel problems.
560	🔴	**Potassium silicate**	A synthetic anti-caking agent. On alert in the United States and the European Union.

570		Stearic acid or Fatty acid	In mass production is a synthetic made from toxic cotton seed oil. Used in dietary supplements. Can cause digestive problems, sensitivity to joints and other health condions.
575		Glucono delta-lactone(GDL) or Gluconolac-tone	Used in commercially made food products and made from glucose. Used for pickling and in many foods. May damage intestinal lining.
576		Sodium gluconate	A synthetic additive used in dietary and nutritional supplements. Also used in baked goods and confectionary. May cause chest pain, buzzing in the ears and other health conditions.
577		Potassium gluconate	A synthetic mineral. Used in many dietary supplements. Can damage intestinal linings. May cause anxiety, confusion and uneven heart beat.

578	●	Calcium gluconate	A synthesized a additive used in meat, pudding powder and other foods. May cause damage to the intestinal lining, heart problems and other health conditions.
579	●	Ferrous gluconate	A food colouring agent used in food supplements. Used in fortified food and baby food. Excessive exposure may lead to enlarged body organs.
580	● ●	Magnesium glucomate	A commercial synthetic used as a flavour enhancer. On alert in the United States, not permitted in the European Union.
586	●	4-Hexyl-resorcinol	Sulphonating benzene, sulphuric acid, caustic soda create benzenedisulfonic acid. Used for long-life shrimp and sea food. May disrupt the endocrine system, linked to cancer.

Devils: Flavour enhancers, glutamates and glutamate boosters (600 range)

620	●	L-glutamic acid	A synthetic bacterial prepared through fermentation dangerous additive. Used as a flavour enhanced and bulking agent in bread, sausages and other foods. Can contribute to eating disorders and other health conditions.
621	●	Monsodium L-glutamate or MSG	A dangerous synthetic derived from bacterial fermentation. Used in sausages, Chinese and Asian meals and other foods. Can cause hyperactivity, ADHD and other health concerns.
622	●	Monopo-tassium L-glutamate	A synthetic prepared from bacterial fermentation. Used in canned tuna, potato chips and other foods. Can cause hypertension, behavioural problems and other health concerns.

623	🔴	Calcium di-L-glutamate	Synthetic bulking agent and bread enhancer. Used in potato chips, stock cubes and other foods. Contributes to hyperactivity, depression and other health problems.
624	🔴	Monoam-monium L-glutamate	Prepared from bacterial fermentation. Used in baked goods, long-life milk and other foods. Contributes to ADHD and health conditions.
625	🔴	Magnesium glutamate	A synthetic additive derived from fermentation of molasses. Used in breads, potato-based snack and other foods. Linked to Alzheimer's and other like illnesses. On alert in the United States.

627	🔴	**Disodium-5'-guanylate also known as: Sodium 5'-guanylate and disodium 5' guanylate**	Extracted from yeast, seaweed and other animal parts. May be genetically modified. Used in rice crackers, macaroni cheese and other foods. Can cause gastrointestinal irritability, headaches and other health problems.
631	🔴	**Disodium-5'-inosinate**	A synthetic additive commercially exploited used in instant noodles, packet soups and other foods. Can trigger gout and related health problems.
635	🔴	**Disodium-5'-ribo-nucleotides**	A synthetic food enhancer used in Chinese food, corn chips and other foods. Can cause gastrointestinal irritability, dizziness and other health conditions. Banned in some countries.
636	🔴	**Maltol**	Commercially, synthetically made. Used in bread, cakes and other foods. Can increase body ability to absorb aluminium.

637	🔴	Ethyl maltol	A synthetic additive which increase the aroma of cooking and cooked bread. Used in the bakery industry. Used in gluten-free bread. Not safe for babies. May cause insomnia. On alert in the United States.
640	🔴	Glycine	Origin of the additive needs to be identified. Used as a food enhancer and bulking agent. Is mildly toxic. See 620.
641	🔴	L-Leucine	Manufactured protein from chemical processes. Used in breads, dietary supplements and other foods. Can cause liver damage, may be toxic. On alert in the European Union.

Devils: Miscellaneous additives (900 range)

900a		Polydimethy-lsiloxane or Dimethyl-polysiloxane (PDMS)	A synthetic, anti-foaming agent added to cooking oils used in the fast-food industry. Can contain formaldehyde. Used in French fries, milk shakes and other fast-foods. Linked to cancer.
901		Beeswax	A natural product. Used in confectionary, ice cream and other foods. May cause allergic reaction.
903		Carnauba wax	Used as a glazing agent in the shine on chocolate production. May cause allergies and possibly a carcinogen.
904		Shellac	A sticky excretion from the Kerria lacca beetle. Used in high-gloss lollies, sweets and other foods. May cause eczema. On alert in the United States.

905	🔴	**Petroleum wax c (i) Micro-crystalline wax (ii) Paraffin wax**	A by-product of petroleum used in dried fruit, confectionary and other foods. May be linked to intestinal disorders and bowel cancer.
905b	🔴	**Petroleum or Petroleum jelly**	A synthesized product made from petroleum products. Used in chocolate, chocolate sweet production and in other foods. May be linked to cancer.
914	🔴	**Oxidised polyethylene**	An ethylene polymer produced from petroleum. Used in glazing in the fruit and vegetable industry. Is linked to cancer.
920	🔴	**L-cysteine mono-hydrochlor-ide**	A synthesized unbound chemical. Used in food supplements, flour and other food products. Linked to endocrine problems
925	🔴	**Chlorine**	A vapour releasing gas, destroys nutrients. Used in tap water. Can cause lung damage. A known carcinogen.

926	●	Chlorine dioxide	Additive derived from urine. Used as a compounding agent to treat flour, used in dough products. Contains formaldehyde. Linked to cancer.
928	● ●	Benzole peroxide	Used as a bleaching agent in white refined flour. May affect asthma sufferers.

Devils: Propellants (900 range)

941	●	Nitrogen	Used for the displacement of moisture in packaging.
942	●	Nitrous oxide	Known as laughing gas. Used in canisters of whipped cream, cooking oils. Can cause headaches and dizziness.
943a	●	Butane	A highly propellant liquid gas and petroleum derivative. Used in aerosol cans for mocked cream and cooking oils. Can contribute to severe allergic reactions.

943b	🔴	Isobutane	A neurotoxic found in spray cans that expel food. May cause headaches, ringing in the ears and other health conditions.
944	🔴	Propane	Is a by-product of petroleum used in aerosol sprays.
946	🟠🔴	Octa-fluoro-cyclobutane or Perfluoro-cyclobutane	Is an aerating agent in food production. More research is required. On alert in the European Union.

Devils: Artificial sweeteners (900 range)

950	🔴	Acesulphame potassium	Highly intensive non-caloric sweetener. Used in frozen desserts, baked food goods and other foods. Is linked to tumours and cancer.
951	🔴	Aspartame Nutrasweet Equal	A synthetic flavour enhancer. Used in jams, breakfast cereals and other foods. Linked to epileptic seizers, depression and other health conditions.

952	●	Cyclamates: (i) Cyclamatic acid (ii) Calcium cyclamate (iii) Potassium cyclamate (iv) Sodium cyclamate	A sulphur trioxide. Used in fizzy drinks, fruit, diet drinks and some cooked food. Can be a carcinogen and contribute to other health conditions.
953	●	Isomalt	A synthetic sweetener used in toffees, cakes and other foods. Is linked to gas, stomach discomfort and other health conditions.
954	●	Saccharins or (i) Saccharin (ii) Calcium Saccharin (iii) Potassium saccharin (iv) Sodium saccharin	A synthetic sweetener. Also extracted from coal tar. Used to sweeten drinks, biscuits and other foods. Is linked to testicular cancer and other healthd conditions. Banned in France, Germany, Hungary, Portugal and Spain.
955	●	Sucralose (Trichloro-galactosucrose)	Is manufactured through chlorinating sugar/sucrose. May cause neurological, immunological damage and weight gain.

956	🔴	**Alitame**	Artificial sweetener at least 2,000 sweeter than sugar. Used in dairy-based drinks, ice cream and other foods. May impair glucose metabolism.
957	🔴	**Thaumatin**	Related to the dangerous additive 620. Used in commercially baked breads, dairy products and other foods. May be responsible for depression, birth defects and other health issues.
960	🟢 🟠	**Steviol glycosides**	A natural product extracted from the plant stevia. Is used in many foods. Methods of extraction need to be known.
961	🟠 🔴	**Neotame**	Is between 7,000 and 13,000 sweeter than sucrose. Used in soft drinks, frozen desserts and other foods. May cause headaches.
962	🔴	**Aspartame-acesulphame salt**	Is highly toxic additive used in dairy shakes, pudding mixes and other foods. Is linked to cancer.

965	○	**Maltitols** (i) Maltitol (ii) Maltitol syrup or Hydrogenated[3] glucose syrup	A sugar alcohol used in low-calorie drinks, baked goods and other foods. More research required. May be linked to birth defects and genetic damage.
966	○ ○	**Lactitol**	A synthetic alcohol used in confectionary, biscuit production and other foods. May contribute to genetic damage. On alert in the United States.
967	○	**Xylitol**	A synthetic alcohol derived from wood pulp. Used in many food products. May cause Irritable Bowel Syndrome (IBS), kidney stones and other health conditions.
968	○	**Erythritol**	Is a sugar alcohol used in low-calorie foods including yogurts, dairy desserts and other foods. May cause bloating and gas. On alert in the United States.

---

[3] To treat with hydrogen through chemical reaction with a catalyst of nickel, palladium or platinum

969		Advantame	Is 20,000 times sweeter than sugar. A synthetic sweetener. Not yet branded. Can be used in high temperature cooking. May have a detrimental effect on gut bacteria.

Devils: Foaming agents (900 range)

999		(i) Quillaia extract (type 1) (ii) Quillaia extract (type 2)	Extracted from the Quillaia saponaria Molina tree. Usually preserved in benzoate or ethanol. Used in frozen dairy desserts, baked goods and other foods. Banned in a number of countries on alert in the United States.

Devils: Additional chemicals and starches

(1001 range)

1001	🔴	Choline salts and esters (i) Choline acetate (ii) Choline carbonate (iii) Choline chloride (iv) Choline citrate (v) Choline tartrate (vi) Choline lactate	Lecithin can be synthetic, if so, may be extracted using hexane. Used in multi-vitamins, sports and other health food products. On alert in the United States, European Union.
1100	🟠	a-Amylase	Derived from mushrooms and pig pancreas. Used in flour and dough products. May be toxic. On alert in the United States and the European Union.
1101	🔴	Proteases (i) Proteases (ii) Papain (iii) Bromelain (iv) Ficin	An enzyme derived from a number of sources. Used as a tenderiser and flavour enhancer for meat; also used in other food sources. On alert in some countries.

1102	🟡 🟠	Glucose oxidase also known as Notatin (GOx)	Used as an additive in dough and bakery products. More research required to justify this additives use in the food industry. . On alert in the United States and the European Union.
1104	🟡 🟠	Lipases	An enzyme widely used in the food industry. Used in margarine, milk chocolate and other food products. More research to justify this additives requirement in the food industry.
1105	🟡 🟠	Lysozyme	Can be genetically modified. May be used in infant food and some hard cheese. May contribute to severe allergic reactions.
1200	🟡	Polydextrose	Is a plasticised mixture of polymer, glucose and sorbitol. Used in manufactured baked foods, jams and other foods. Not to be given to infants.

1201	🔴	**Polyviny-lpyrrolidone PVP**	Produced from formaldehyde, acetylene, hydrogen and ammonia. Used in low-joule foods, white wine and other food or drink products. May cause intestinal blockage, cancer and other health problems.
1400	🟠 🔴	**Dextrin roasted starch**	Not fully researched. Used in gluten-free foods, bakery, batters and other food products. Look for chemicals. May be used in baby food. On alert in the European Union.
1401	🟠 🔴	**Acid treated starch**	Used as a thickening agent. Is gluten-free. Used in commercial pizzas, French dressing and other food products. On alert in the United States.

1402	🟡 🟠	**Alkaline treated and modified starch. Also known as Lye or costic soda**	Used as a thickening agent. Also used commercially in pizzas, frozen foods and other food products. More research required. On alert in the United States and other countries
1403	🟠	**Bleached starch**	A modified enzyme bleached with sulphur dioxide. Used as a thickening agent in custards, baby formulas and other food. Not fully evaluated. On alert in the United States and the European Union.
1404	🟠	**Oxidised starch**	Used as a thickening agent. Added to jellies, yogurts and other foods and confectionary. Is linked to cancer, kidney and liver disorders. On alert in the United States. Not approved in the European Union.

1410	🔴	**Monostarch phosphate**	Used as a thickener, may be bleached. Used in some baby foods, puddings and other foods. Linked to high cholesterol and other health conditions. See 1410. More research on the product is required. On alert in the United States.
1412	🔴	**Distarch phosphate**	Used as a thickening agent in baby foods, batter mixes, ice cream and other foods. May contribute to pathological changes in the lungs. Further research and evaluation required. On alert in the United States.
1413	🔴	**Phosphated distarch phosphate**	A synthetic additive, possibly made from genetically modified starch. Used in jelly-based sweets, cola drinks and other foods and drinks. Is linked to high blood cholesterol, kidney and stomach disorder. On alert in the United States.

1414	🔴	**Acetylated distarch phosphate**	A synthetic thickening agent used in many industries. Used in baby food, batter mixes and other foods. May contribute to cancer, high blood cholesterol and other health related conditions. Dangerous for asthmatics. On alert in the United States.
1420	🔴	**Starch acetate**	Used as a thickener, which may be bleached. Used in yogurts, some baby foods and other foods and confectionary. Dangerous for asthmatics, may leave calcium deposits in the kidneys. On alert in the United States.
1422	🔴	**Acetylated distarch adipate**	Can be genetically modified. Used in baby foods, take away foods and other food products. Is a cancer proven chemical. Further testing is required. On alert in the United States.

1440	●	**Hydroxypropyl starch**	Is a food stabiliser which may be produced from genetically modified grain. Used in yogurt, ice cream and other commercially made foods. On alert in the United States.
1442	●	**Hydroxypropyl distarch phosphate**	A food stabiliser and thickener. Used in ice cream, microwave noodles and other foods. Linked to calcium deposits in the kidneys and other health concerns. On alert in the United States.
1450	●	**Starch sodium octenylsuccin-ate**	Is a food thickener possibly derived from genetically modified grain. Used in long-life milk, baby food and other foods. Proven cancer causing chemicals. On alert in the United States.

1451	🔴	Acetylated oxidised starch	A synthetic widely used in the food industry. Used in baby food, jelly-based sweets and in a wide range of foods. Can contribute to pathological changes in the lungs, linked to cancer and other health conditions.
1505	🔴	Triethyl citrate	Commercially produced from citric acid. Used in sports drinks, egg whites and in other foods. See 620, contains PFGA. Has the ability to interfere with the human brain.
1518	🔴	Triacetin	Manufactured through chemical process from glycerol. Is a plasticizer and solvent used in many industries. Used to coat fresh fruit and vegetables. Is a neurotoxin.

1520	🔴	Propylene glycol or 1,2-propane-diol 1,2-dihydr-oxy propane Methyl ethy-lene glycol Propane-1,2-diol and brand names	Is a synthetic, petroleum-based compound used to maximise shelf-life in many foods. Is a humectant. Used in chocolate, hot chilli sauce and other foods. May contributes to depression, fatal heart attacks and other health conditions.
1521	🔴	Polyethylene glycol 8000 1,2-propane diol 1,2-dihydroxy propane Methyl ethylene glycol Propane-1,2-diol and brand names	Is petroleum based, synthesized from urea and propylene glycol. Is used as a bread enhancer. Use in chocolate-based confectionary. Is linked to depression, cancer and other health conditions.
1522	🔴	Calcium lignosulphonate (40-65)	Synthetic alcohols from softwood. Used as a fat carrier in vitamins, dairy products and other foods. Further research required. On alert in the European Union. For further reading on this additive, please see Devils in our Food.

80

Devils in Our Food and App also available at:

www.how2books.com.au

See
Devils In Our Food

For a full description
of food additives.

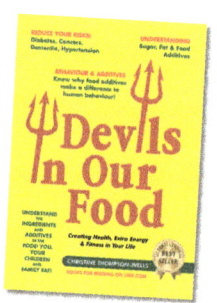

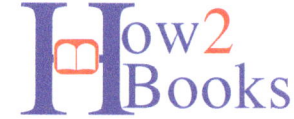

www.how2books.com.au

> Food awareness can reduce health problems, limit pain and increase life's abundance.

www.ingramcontent.com/pod-product-compliance
Lightning Source LLC
Chambersburg PA
CBHW062042290426
44109CB00026B/2705